Eat for Energy the Glycemic Index Way

Boost Energy Levels Without the Insulin Spikes

RON KNESS

Contents

Disclaimer

This publication is for informational purposes only and is not intended as medical advice. Medical advice should always be obtained from a qualified medical professional for any health conditions or symptoms associated with them.

Every possible effort has been made in preparing and researching this material. We make no warranties with respect to the accuracy, applicability of its contents or any omissions.

See your healthcare professional before starting any diet or exercise program!

Introduction

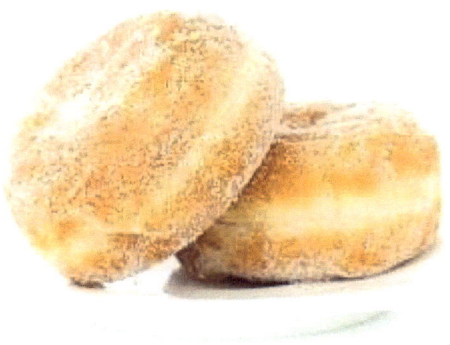

In this book, we are exploring the connection between what you eat and the energy you have throughout the day. One of the major factors that can be used in eating for energy is the Glycemic Index (GI). Nutrition and fitness coaches have been talking about the glycemic index for a while, and this talk has created a buzz among ordinary people who just want to be healthy.

If you are not familiar with the Glycemic Index, it is a numerical value assigned to different sources of carbohydrates. As you might have heard, carbs are not created the same. Some are good. Others not so much.

It's just that our digestive system isn't built to handle all carbs the same way. While it digests simple carbohydrates like sugars fast, it takes longer to break down complex carbohydrates, such as whole grain. The length of time it takes your gut to break down carbs affects the rate at which your glucose level rises after your meal.

It is called the glycemic response. Your body converts carbs and sugars to glucose, the simplest form of carbohydrate that your cells can use as fuel.

Glycemic index is basically a scale from 0 to 100. Lower values means conversion to glucose happens slowly. Higher values more quickly. In other words, foods with high glycemic index are quickly turned to glucose and cause a quick rise in your blood glucose level. Foods with low GI are the opposite, of course.

Dr. David Jenkins and his associates were noted for their work on this crucial data in nutritional science. Various studies have been done so far to test the effects of different types of carbohydrates in terms of glycemic index. Factors examined include the rate of glucose rise and the insulin response. Long-term studies involve effects of high glycemic index carbs in the long run. What scientists found out are crucial in developing diet modifications to preclude diabetes.

As noted before, generally simple sugars have high GI. Your digestive system quickly turns them into glucose. Glucose then gets passed into the bloodstream. In turn, your blood glucose levels rise and stimulates your pancreas to release insulin. This hormone, as we know, is the transporter and is what is responsible for moving glucose into cells. The cells use it as their source of energy so that they can function. However, excess glucose may be turned into glycogen and deposited in the adipose tissue.

Complex carbohydrates mostly have low GI. Your stomach and small intestines take a longer time to break them down into glucose. As a result, glucose gets passed into the bloodstream at a slower rate. Voila! No glucose and insulin spikes.

Understanding these simple principles of carbohydrate digestion, glucose rate absorption, and insulin response is a key to making healthier food choices. The human body is designed to tolerate only a narrow range of glucose levels. That means it is imperative you keep your sugar levels within this normal range. You don't want your blood sugar to drop too low, because you would suffer from hypoglycemia. You also don't want it to become too high.

Bad food choices raises your risk for a number of conditions, such as reactive hypoglycemia and type 2 diabetes.

Earlier, we touched on reactive hypoglycemia lightly. It happens when your blood sugar becomes too high immediately after a meal. During this sugar spike, you feel good and energetic. Insulin then rushes in as a response. This causes your glucose to drop just as fast as it rose. So now you feel sluggish and hungry. However, unchecked rapid decline of your blood sugar puts your body in a state of emergency. Your stress hormones (cortisol, epinephrine, and norepinephrine) are released.

Experts think that reactive hypoglycemia isn't bad on its own. It's the activation of stress hormones that causes the classic symptoms of hypoglycemia. These symptoms include fatigue, shakiness, sweating, and heart palpitations.

Reactive hypoglycemia can occur due to a number of reasons, but it can happen due to diets rich in simple sugars. It's a warning sign that you have to modify your diet. Shifting to complex carbohydrates is one way to avoid drastic shifts in the concentration of glucose in your blood, thus precluding wild insulin response, the sudden drop in glucose concentrations, and the stress hormone release that happens afterwards.

Diets high in simple sugars pose another threat, a more common one. Type 2 diabetes is rising in incidence due to poor diet and lifestyle choices. It's not just the sudden rise in blood sugar you should be worried about. It's the long term effect of frequent elevations of your sugar levels, which happens in diets composed of foods with high glycemic index. At some point, your body starts to resist insulin. So insulin is no longer able to transport glucose into the cells. It stays in your bloodstream to keep your blood sugar levels above normal.

Of course, these are simplistic explanations, but the point is, making better food choices is a key to good health and wellness. But how can you make good choices when you don't know what the good choices are?

Carb Intake and Energy Levels

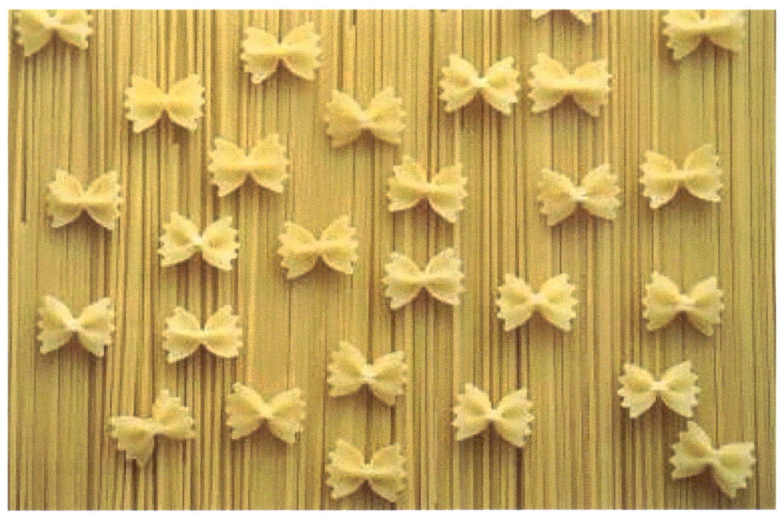

Half of the daily calories you consume each day should come from carbohydrates. The other half should be split between protein at 30% and healthy fats at 20%. But those are only starting points. To fine your intake, the carbohydrate range can be 45-65% according to the Dietary Guidelines for Americans. For a 2,000 calories a day diet, 900-1,300 of those calories should come from carbs.

Does this mean you have to start counting your calories?

If you're worried about your weight or about your calorie intake in general, you may consider counting your calories. It's not as hard as you think. Packaged food contains nutrition labels, which includes calories per serving. However, be sure to note how many servings are in a package. You may think it is one, when in fact it is more. You can also Google nutrition facts of the foods you are consuming. The info is just a few mouse clicks away.

Carbs are your main energy source.

A lot of self-proclaimed nutrition experts have demonized carbs in favor of the other two macronutrients fats and protein. The thing is, you need all three in varying amounts. There is no good and evil when it comes to nutrients. The most important reason carbohydrates are considered a macronutrient is because a huge bulk of your meal should comprise them. As noted before, roughly half of your meal should be carbs. Protein isn't your body's chief source of energy. It has other more important functions; the same is true with fat.

It doesn't matter what else you have heard or read. Glucose is the chief source of energy. The main question for a lot of fitness buffs is how much glucose is necessary. There is no definite answer. It varies from person to person. It depends on your daily energy requirements, which in turn depends on your lifestyle, occupation, and fitness levels. What we know is if you eat less than your total daily energy requirement for a period of time, you'll shed off weight. You gain when you eat more than that.

Energy requirements are arbitrary.

There are different kinds of people. There's the office guy; there's the athlete; there's the average gym guy. People who lift weights or run marathons burn more calories than the office guy. So the first thing you have to look into is your daily activity. What do you do during the whole course of the day? If you spend much of your time on your feet, moving about, and if you sweat a lot, lifting weights, you're better off on high-carb diet. If you spend much of the day sitting down, doing lightweight activities, you're better off on a low-carb diet.

To maintain your current weight, the principle is simple - eat only the amount of calories your body needs on a daily basis.

But what if you want to gain muscle?

Building muscle requires intense workouts. Lifting weights in the gym requires a different source of energy. The amount of free glucose coursing through your body isn't enough when you're tearing your muscle fibers apart in the gym. Much of the time, your body has to tap into energy reserves. That's where glycogen comes in. People who constantly work out, those who have daily fitness routines, need to have ample supply of glycogen in their livers and muscles. Glycogen is your important energy source when you're doing intense exercise. Maintaining a good supply of it is a key to enhanced workout performance.

Several studies have already mentioned that high-carbohydrate diets are beneficial for muscle growth than low-carbohydrate diets. A few things happen when you're on a high-carb diet. You have more energy reserves, so you perform better on your workouts. You have energy left over after a workout, so you don't suffer from post-workout fatigue. Your insulin rises, creating an environment that promotes muscle growth. Also, take note that muscle repair happens at the expense of energy, which is what they refer to as the after burn.

You know what they say at the gym: you need caloric surplus when you want to build muscle. That surplus is provided by extra carbs. It's not just protein you need to increase in amount if you're looking to build muscle, but also your carb intake.

Muscle gains can't occur on a low-carb diet. Your body will look for other sources of energy, and that's when protein breakdown happens. Serious carb depletion results in breakdown of muscle. That is counterproductive.

How much carbs should you eat then if you want to gain muscle? Depending on your activity levels and the intensity of your workouts, you need 1-3 grams of carbohydrates per pound of body weight.

What if you want to lose fat?

You may think it's reasonable to drop the cups of brown rice and go on a low-carb crusade. However, if we are to look at the results of low-carb diets on fat loss, the findings are surprising. Unless you're obese, you don't need to go on a low-carb diet. In many cases, a diet that's low on something doesn't work. You need to check and maybe tweak your portions, making sure you get enough of all the macros and you're on slight caloric deficit – generally ingesting about 500 fewer calories per day then what you burn. Drastic reductions in carbs are counterproductive if weight loss is your goal.

Why Complex Carbs are Better

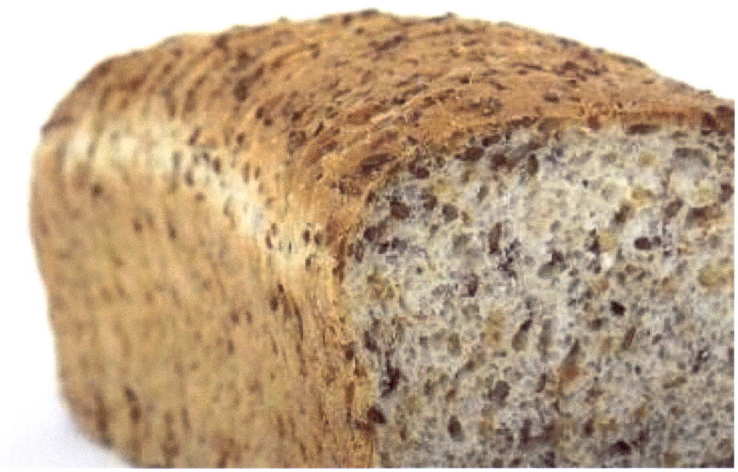

You probably heard people saying eat oats or whole grain bread instead of this and that. At some point you found the whole diet planning irksome because you have to keep in mind a lot of things. Don't fret. You will eventually get used to it, and you'll realize making the right choices isn't as difficult as you think.

Perhaps it's all right to learn a bit about what happens when you eat carbs. The role of your digestive system is to break down what you eat (except most fiber). Your digestive system breaks down carbohydrates into a form every cell in your body can use - glucose. It's the source of energy. Your cells are programmed to use glucose to do their work.

But the story doesn't end there. As your digestive system breaks down carbohydrates and introduces glucose into your bloodstream, your blood glucose levels rise.

Unfortunately, your cells cannot absorb the glucose on their own. They need a transport device which is where insulin comes in. It is the hormone that gets the glucose in your bloodstream into your cells where it can be used for energy.

As your glucose levels rise after your meal, your pancreas releases insulin to help move glucose into cells. As glucose is moved into your cells, your glucose levels fall as a result. This decrease in blood sugar prompts the pancreas to release another hormone, glucagon. This hormone tells your liver to release stored sugar. These mechanisms ensure your body's steady supply of glucose and thus ensure you have energy throughout the day.

What you just read may not seem like crucial information. After all, it's what your body does. It's automatic. It's preprogrammed. That's true to some extent. People with type 2 diabetes know their bodies can take only so much. After years of poor diet and lifestyle choices, your body may develop resistance to insulin. As a result, glucose no longer gets into cells and stays in the blood. Glucose-depleted cells cannot function properly, and one of the telltale signs of this is fatigue, a common symptom of diabetes.

But this book is not directly about diabetes. Instead, it is about the crucial mechanisms involved in the cascade of events that happen inside your body after you eat. These dips and spikes in glucose occur as many times as you eat. But how much your sugar rises and falls depends on a number of things. One is the kind of carbohydrates you're eating.

As we said before, not all carbohydrates are built the same. The differences in the molecular structures of many carbohydrates mean that some carbs are digested faster than the others. It doesn't seem like a big deal, but how fast your glucose levels rise depends on how fast your carbs are being digested. Simple carbohydrates tend to be digested faster. Complex carbohydrates tend to be digested slower. Simple carbs, thus, cause rapid rise in glucose levels after a meal.

But so what if your glucose rises fast after a meal?

Ideally, you want your body to introduce glucose slowly into the cells so that its concentration in the blood doesn't plummet. The thing is, your body doesn't do that. It can't control the absorption of too much glucose in the bloodstream into the cells. What happens is, the pancreas simply releases too much insulin to compensate for the amount of sugar in the bloodstream. Then glucose is fed into the cells quickly because of all the insulin in your bloodstream to take it inside the cells. This causes a spike in energy levels. But the spike in insulin rapidly depletes your glucose reserves. Thus, you feel the drop in energy soon after.

These wild fluctuations of sugar levels create fluctuations in energy and mood throughout the day, and the average person does not realize it. So this is what happens. You eat a bowl of cornflakes in the morning and feel good until 10 a.m. After that, you feel hungry. You're running low on sugar now, and your brain is telling you to go grab something to eat, preferably sweet. The likely scenarios are, one, you grab snacks or a bagel or cinnamon roll or two, you overeat at lunch. Then the cycle happens again.

Your sugar spikes for an hour or two, and then you feel sleepy, irritable, and hungry in the middle afternoon. It's a vicious cycle that wreaks havoc to your body over time.

Your goal is to keep your sugar levels stable throughout the day. Eating the right kind of carbohydrates at the right time fixes the issue. Complex carbs generally have low glycemic index. Your digestive system takes a while to break them down, so glucose gets released in a steady stream rather than in a huge bulk at once. With complex carbs, you get a steady supply of glucose, and you don't go through drastic fluctuations in your sugar levels. Your insulin doesn't fluctuate dramatically as well, and you don't get as great of a stress hormone response, which is the real culprit.

How Simple Sugars Affect Glucose Levels

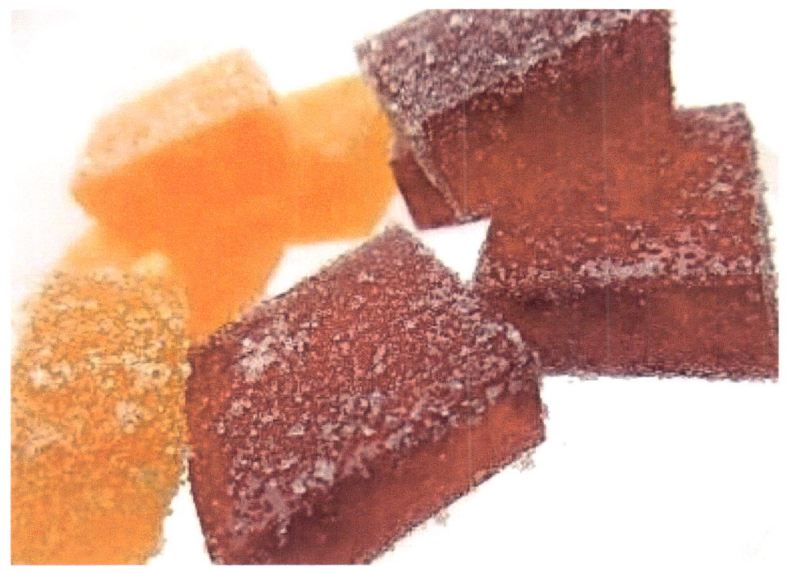

It would have been a happy life if you could just eat anything and not worry about getting fat or having to fill your prescriptions for metformin 5 years later. But that's just not the case. As much as you want to indulge in everything, it's just not possible to eat what you want and not suffer the consequences of poor diet choices. And simple sugars are one of the most frequently consumed unhealthy foods.

You probably put sugar in your coffee or glaze your toast with something high in sugar like jelly or jam. Sugar is everywhere. It's in your ice cream. It's in milk. It's in chocolate drinks. It's in soda. It's in a lot of things that you like, things you're supposed to consume sparingly, but actually consume frequently.

It's easy to grab a slice of cake or two. It's easy to help yourself to cinnamon rolls when you're hungry. You crave sweets when you're sad or sleep deprived. You grab a can of soda when you're thirsty.

It's not so bad. After all, you're just hungry. After all, it's just carbs. And, hey, who doesn't need carbs? Carbs are for energy.

Not so fast!

Carbs aren't built the same. One is different from another. White bread isn't nutritionally similar to wholegrain bread. Corn isn't the same as cornflakes. Brown rice is different from white rice. These are crucial differences in terms of nutrient value, glycemic index and ultimately how fast your body processes each one.

Simple sugars generally have high glycemic index. They have simple structures, so your digestive system quickly breaks them down to glucose. You don't have to be a genius to understand that it's easier to break down simpler things than complex things.

The following events happen:

- Your glucose levels shoot up.

- Insulin rushes in. It's actually an insulin spike.

- Cells take in glucose.

- Glucose is either used for energy or stored as glycogen.

- Your glucose levels plunge.

If you have two or more meals a day, and these meals include simple sugars, you're bound to have wild fluctuations of glucose throughout the day. You're also bound to experience insulin spikes and energy spikes and dips throughout the day.

Of course, there are other factors that may cause sugar and insulin spikes in your blood, and if you're suffering from these maladies, you need to seriously look into your diet choices and your health in general.

But what's the big deal? Well, your energy level depends on how much glucose you have in your system. Your cells look for free glucose in your blood for energy. If you don't have enough of it, your body will look for it somewhere. Your pancreas releases glucagon, which causes the liver to release stored glycogen. But this process isn't supposed to happen frequently. It's not about the frequent release of glucagon per se. It's about what else your body goes through when it runs low of sugar. It enters a stress mode, something your body doesn't need frequently and takes its toll eventually.

Your body only works within a narrow range of glucose levels (70-110 mg/dL). Your goal should be to keep your glucose levels within this range so as not to put stress on your vital organs -- for instance, your pancreas. Because at some point the mechanisms involved in stabilizing your blood sugar levels -- the complex interaction between insulin and glucagon (as well as other hormones like epinephrine and cortisol) -- will succumb to frequent spikes in your glucose levels.

People who suffer from reactive hypoglycemia can attest to this. They feel good after a sugary meal. Three hours later they feel lethargic, dizzy, short of breath, and confused -- the evil signs of hypoglycemia, the ironic downside of having too much sugar in your bloodstream. Sure, you sip some soda or grab a piece of hard candy. It gives short term relief. But a healthy diet rich in complex carbs ought to keep this condition from bothering you in the first place.

Breakfasts That Provide Energy All Day

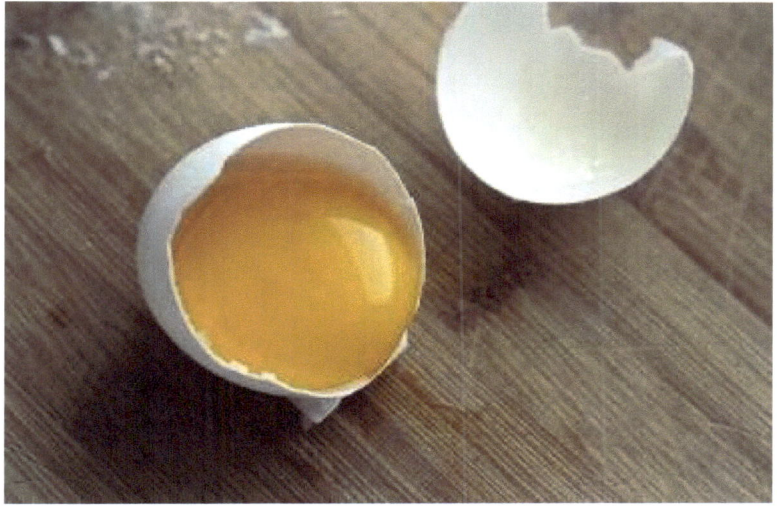

Breakfast may or may not be your most important meal of the day, but skipping it isn't always a good idea. It's all right to start your day with a good meal, unless you're doing intermittent fasting, which studies have shown to be not really more effective than eating a healthy diet. It's a good way to kick start your metabolism after your body has been fasting for the last 8 hours or so.

The purpose of breakfast is to fill your body with the nutrients it needs to get you up and running in the morning and to keep you going until lunch. You haven't eaten anything since dinner last night, and your body is low on glucose. If you don't eat anything in the morning, your body will take calories from elsewhere. Your liver will release glycogen. You may even burn fat or muscle.

The question is, what should you eat in the morning?

You can just eat anything, and get away with it if you're young. After all, I used to eat chocolate cake for breakfast occasionally when I was young. (True!)

But bad diet habits often show their evil heads when you're older (and that is also true as I'm now finding out!). But it's never too late to choose healthier breakfasts for a healthier you.

Avoid simple carbs and processed food!

That advice is like the holy grail of dieting. It's something you have to keep in mind, especially if you want to lead a healthy life. Processed food is rich in simple sugars and sweeteners, too, that do just the same. They also contain junk (i.e. preservatives), which your body doesn't need and actually shouldn't have.

Making healthy breakfast should be your goal, and it's possible by choosing complex carbs and protein-rich foods.

Oatmeal. This isn't a fad. Healthy people eat oatmeal for a number of reasons. Two of the most important are oatmeal's glycemic index and its fiber content. It doesn't taste good by itself, but being a complex carbohydrate and being rich in fiber, make it your morning best friend. A lot of people complain about its taste good, but this is easily remedied by adding some walnuts or fresh fruit, such as blueberries as mentioned later in this chapter. A slice of mango too can add taste to an otherwise dull breakfast. Some people like oatmeal served with milk. Personally, I use Silk® Almond Milk that has 0 grams of sugar, but tastes great.

Bananas. Health buffs don't add a banana with their cereal for nothing. Bananas are rich in potassium, among other things. But potassium, which helps you lower your blood pressure, is what makes it a popular choice among dieters and health-conscious eaters. Bananas are handy. You can make smoothies out of them. Smoothies for breakfast are becoming a popular choice among busy professionals who still want to stay fit, but you are better off making your own instead of buying them pre-made as many are high in added sugar. To top it all, bananas have low glycemic index. It's not going to cause your sugar to suddenly shoot up.

Eggs. Eggs have been demonized for being rich in cholesterol. The yolks are rich in cholesterol, but they're also rich in choline, vitamin B-complex, and vitamin D. Besides, several studies have shown dietary cholesterol has no effect on your blood cholesterol. Your liver is doing fine keeping your blood cholesterol levels within healthy levels, unless it's not working properly. You shouldn't stay away from eggs; two per day won't hurt you at all. They're good for your brain. Their protein content is good for your muscles and will keep your energy levels up throughout the day.

Whole-wheat bread. It contains more nutrients and fiber than white bread. In the food department, white means something has been processed. White bread has higher glycemic index than wholegrain or whole-wheat bread. You probably won't eat whole-wheat bread alone. Slather almond butter on your bread to get protein. You can also eat it with eggs – eggs and a piece of wholegrain toast make a great breakfast. Or for lunch, you could make a sandwich with lettuce, tomatoes, and egg. Look for the whole grain stamp on the package.

Cereal. Choose the right one. Something with at least 5 grams of fiber and less than 5 grams of sugar is good. Whole-grain cereal is your best bet. It's rich in folic acid, B vitamins, and other minerals. Served with milk, it's perfect, especially if you don't have time to prepare breakfast.

Blueberries. These nutrient-packed fruits are rich in antioxidants. With all their nutrient combo, they do a lot of things, like lower your blood pressure and improve your metabolism. They're considered a superfood because they're nutrient dense and pack few calories.

Smart Eating Habits

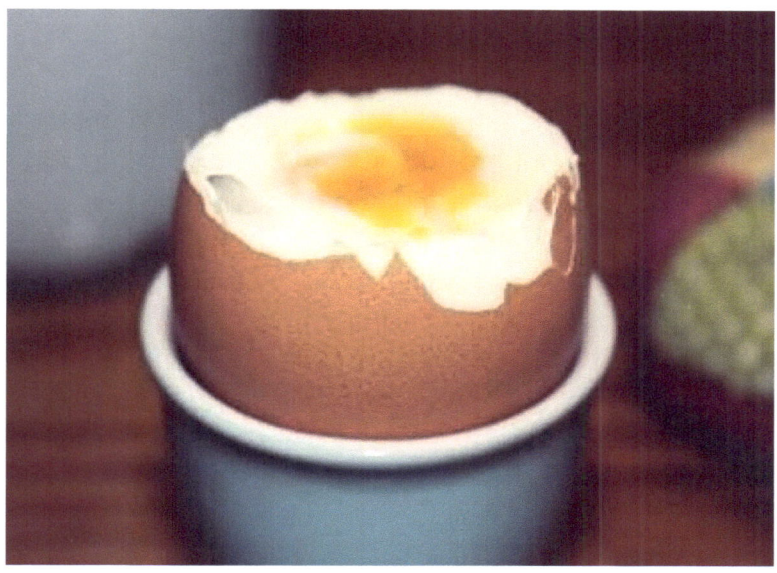

What and how you eat affect your mood, alertness, and performance throughout the day. A lot of people don't realize this fact. They attribute their mood swings and performance decline as the day wanes to stress but fail to see the impact of their diet on their ability to function well. If you feel spirited and alert in the morning but don't feel the same way in the afternoon, you probably need to look at your eating habits and make changes.

Eat a satisfying breakfast.

Most people eat a light breakfast. Maybe a bagel or a sandwich will do. They drink their coffee, and off they go.

Morning is when you're supposed to have a good meal, not a light one, especially after spending the night under the sheets on empty stomach. It's when you're supposed to replenish your body of the macronutrients, vitamins, and minerals to jump start your day.

Unfortunately, people either don't eat breakfast or they eat an unhealthy one, but they overeat at dinner. This is bad because your body doesn't have the time before you go to bed to digest the calories you consumed during that late meal.

Serve protein in the morning.

A satisfying breakfast needs to include protein. Maybe serve hard-boiled eggs, quinoa, beans, or chicken (minus the skin). Protein delays the digestion of everything you eat, including carbohydrates. If you eat white rice (better yet brown rice) with chicken, the protein in chicken slows down the digestion of rice. In so doing, it helps slow down the passage of glucose into the blood. But what's the big deal?

Does the following scenario sound familiar? You eat a bagel and drink your coffee at 7 o'clock in the morning. You go to work, and around 10 o'clock you start yawning. You start feeling a little hazy. You lose concentration. You feel hungry. You leave your desk, head to the cafeteria, and buy some cinnamon roll or muffins.

Nope, you're not just feeling hungry. It's probably not just job stress. The bagel and coffee you had for breakfast sabotaged your energy levels. Bagel has simple carbs that easily get digested and turned into glucose, raising your blood sugar.

Coupled with caffeine in your coffee, it gives you that temporary energy boost, which lasts for two or three hours, after which your brain starts telling you to grab something else to eat.

It's a vicious cycle that can be prevented by slowing down the digestion of carbs. One way is by adding protein in your meals.

Eat whole grains.

Whole grains have not been processed or refined, and so they have higher fiber content and have retained much of their nutrient content. It takes a longer time for them to be digested than refined grains. That's why they're considered low GI foods. Again, this is about stabilizing your glucose levels as much as possible. You're better off having your energy levels stable throughout the day than having drastic swings in your glucose and insulin levels. Like protein, low GI carbs help you feel fuller longer and thus keeps the hunger in between meals away.

Avoid white bread, bagels, cinnamon rolls, fruit juices, and anything sweet and made with white refined flour.

Nix the coffee.

Caffeine in coffee is the silent evil. It perks you up, but lets you down. It's a mild stimulant with addictive properties. It taxes your adrenal glands, releasing stress hormones that keep you on the go for a brief period, after which you start trailing off. It's your dishonest best friend, one that fires you up but uses up your resources and leaves you empty and downtrodden. Don't let its lure deceive you.

There are two ways to get rid of caffeine. One is by stopping right away, which gives you nasty headaches and drowsiness. Another is by stopping gradually, which is manageable for most. When you're experiencing the unpleasant signs of adrenal fatigue, you'll realize the need to give up your espresso and latte.

Eat several small meals.

Large meals also cause wild sugar spikes and dips. To avoid this, eat five or six smaller meals throughout the day. Just ensure you are not eating more calories than you should – small means small. For example, if you are on an 1,800 calories per day diet and have six small meals per day, each meal would be around 300 calories.

Small meals raise your blood sugar levels just a little, and when you're glucose is on the downhill road, go grab another small meal. Don't just eat anything, though. Make sure you're eating meals rich in protein, low GI carbs, and fiber. Choices don't have to be difficult. Think of eggs, tuna, wholegrain bread, almond butter, and apples. Also, snacking on nuts isn't a bad idea. The point is to keep your bloodstream glucose at a fairly steady rate.

The Fiber Connection

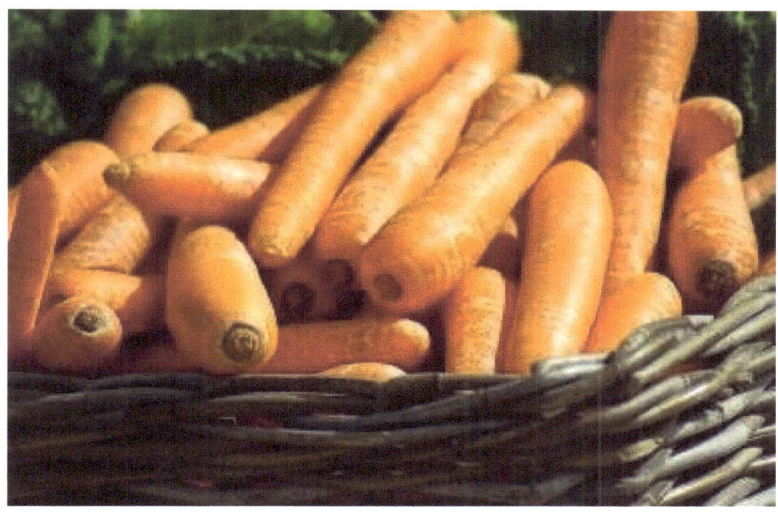

Fiber is actually a type of carbohydrate and comes as soluble and insoluble. Insoluble is the type your digestive system cannot break down. That seems to tell us that type of fiber is useless, but our body's inability to digest it is actually its advantage.

What is fiber?

It's the component of grains, nuts, beans, vegetables, and fruits that the humans cannot digest. Hence, most of it enters and exits your body undigested. Because it cannot be digested, it acts like a cleaner, sweeping your gastrointestinal tract as it moves along and carries the sludge with it.

What are the health benefits of fiber?

One of the oldest known health benefit of fiber is it facilitates normal bowel movement. Much of your stools is made up of fiber, which carries with it waste material in your digestive tract. By keeping your bowel movement healthy, you are reducing your risk of constipation and also reduces your risk of diverticulitis and hemorrhoids.

Fiber also lowers your bad LDL cholesterol, thus reducing your risk of heart disease and stroke. It also lowers your risk of diabetes because it retards the absorption of sugar and stabilizes your blood sugar levels.

Can fiber give you more energy?

It can't. Your body cannot break it down like it can break down regular carbs. So it cannot give you energy. It doesn't get any simpler than that.

So how can it give you more energy?

It seems counterintuitive to eat something for energy if your body cannot convert it to something that provides energy. But that's not the point. The effects of fiber on your energy levels has something to do with its role in digestion.

Let's talk about the glycemic index first.

These are two words you have heard before, but have to remember when you encounter carbohydrates. As noted before, the glycemic index (GI) is determined by how fast a type of carbohydrate is digested. As a review, high GI foods tend to be broken down faster than low GI foods. Because of that, high GI foods introduce glucose faster into your bloodstream than low GI foods.

In turn, the former causes your glucose to rise faster than the latter.

So looks like high GI foods can provide you with more energy? Within a short period. But high glucose in the blood after eating cake or bagel prompts the pancreas to release insulin and shelves glucose into the cells. You're left with low blood sugar after this. High GI foods cause fluctuations, thereby putting your body on stress. That's why health advocates recommend complex carbs, which generally have low GI.

So where does fiber enter the picture?

The idea of glycemic index is simplistic. You can say oatmeal has low GI and cinnamon rolls have high GI. White rice has higher GI than brown rice. But we don't eat white rice alone, for instance. We usually pair it with veggies or beans (or chicken or fish). What you eat your carbs with affects the overall glycemic index of your meal. How about getting the best of both worlds and eat your pairing with brown rice instead of white!

If you pair white rice with veggies or lentils (of course, you'll also have your protein, like salmon or chicken), you're increasing the fiber content of your meal. Fiber retards the digestion of carbohydrates and lowers the glycemic index of your meal. This is one of the reasons why you should include fiber in your diet.

As fiber slows down the breakdown of carbohydrates, it also slows down the absorption of glucose into the blood. Your body then receives glucose at a steadier rate than it otherwise would if you didn't eat fiber. A steady supply of glucose ensures you have stable energy throughout the day.

You don't suffer from sugar spike and crash, which is associated with high GI food.

How much fiber should you eat?

The recommended daily intake is 20-35 grams. Most people, however, get only half of that. That is not good news, especially when you look at data of rising cases of type 2 diabetes. Increasing your fiber intake isn't so hard. Adding wholegrain food, vegetables, fruits, and legumes to your diet raises your dietary fiber intake. If you can't prepare your food and you eat at restaurants, order oatmeal, nuts, or salad, instead of potato chips and cornflakes.

How Easily Digestible Foods Provide More Energy

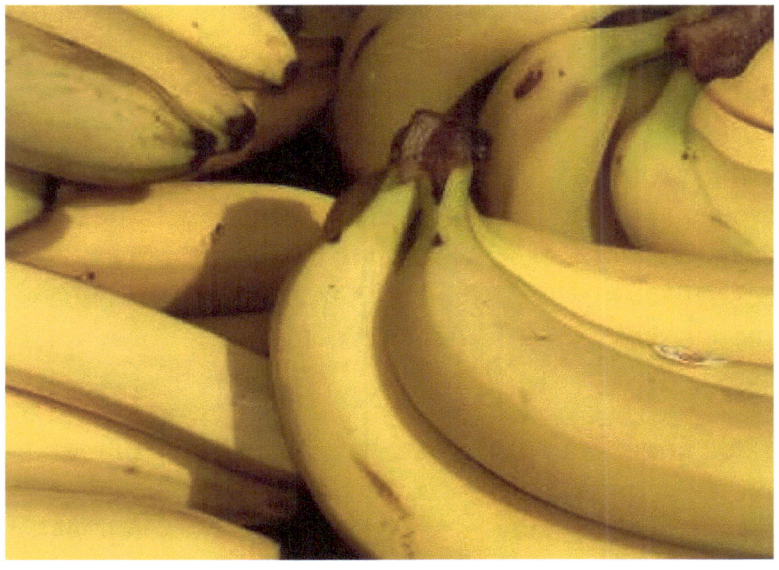

Should you be only eating complex carbs and disregarding simple carbs altogether?

Energy comes from food. You cannot get it anywhere else. Different types of food provide different amounts of energy. Among the three macronutrients carbs, protein, and fat, your best bet for energy is carbs. Both protein and healthy fats have more important functions than to provide energy. Yes, it's carbohydrates that mainly fuels you throughout the day. Your body turns carbs to glucose and uses it to fuel cellular activity, basically fueling all your body's functions and activities. Carbs chief role is to fuel you.

But there are different types of carbs.

Health buffs often say that complex carbs are the way to go. They take a long time to break down, so they don't turn to glucose right away. This is a good thing because rapid conversion of carbs to glucose causes sugar spikes. It's not the sugar spike on its own that's detrimental. In fact, the sudden influx of glucose in your body makes a lot of people feel good. What comes after is the problem. Too much insulin is produced. It kicks in and sends the glucose into your cells. It doesn't sound bad, except that your body activates its stress response when it runs low of free glucose. It's a nasty business associated with a combo of hormones that tell your liver it's time to break down glycogen.

You don't need that dramatic interaction among different hormones in your body. You don't need dramatic sugar fluctuations. Your body is designed to handle sugar within a narrow concentration range. Outside that range, your system just runs amok.

Also, a diet rich in simple carbs raises your risk of type 2 diabetes. Doctors never recommend simple sugars to pre-diabetics and diabetics because they already have elevated sugar levels. Sudden rise in sugar levels is adding fuel to the fire.

However, there are instances when simple carbs are especially needed.

There are instances wherein fast breakdown of carbs and absorption of glucose into the blood are just the things you need. The most common instance wherein you need to quickly raise your glucose level is right after a strenuous activity (e.g. weight training or marathon).

Exercise uses up the glucose in your blood. It's one of the most effective ways to reduce your blood sugar. That is why it's highly recommended for diabetics. Strenuous workouts, however, can deplete your body of glucose. By the end of your activity, your sugar level is probably too low. Your muscles may have depleted their glycogen.

Replenishing your glycogen stores is important after your workout. Muscle growth does not only require protein but also glycogen. You need to replenish lost glycogen right away. This is why post-workout meals include protein shakes and simple carbs. Notice that these are easily digestible foods. The goal is to replenish lost fuel during heavy physical activity as fast as possible. Your muscles need protein to rebuild torn muscle fibers. They also need their glycogen stores refilled.

There's another important reason why you should eat quick-to-digest foods after heavy workout. These foods keep your sugar from plummeting further after it has been depleted during your workout. Not eating anything after intense training increases chances of hypoglycemia, a condition wherein your blood sugar drops below normal. In extreme cases, it can be life-threatening.

Just as you don't want your sugar too high, you also don't want it too low because your brain and body suffer. If you suddenly feel lethargic and shaky after your workout, you could be suffering from low blood sugar. That signals you to eat simple carbs to replenish used up glucose. You can't spend a long time on empty stomach after your workout. Doing so negatively affects your muscle gains and your available energy for post-workout activities.

Marathon runners, on the other hand, do what we call carb-loading. This is only applicable for endurance athletes. The average person shouldn't do it. Carb-loading, as its name implies, means loading up on carbs two or three days before a marathon. The diet is heavily composed of carbs. We're talking 90% of food on the plate. Much of the carbs are high GI carbs, such as bagel and fruits. The goal is to amp up glycogen stores to provide enough fuel to carry one through a marathon.

Should You Turn to Fat for Energy?

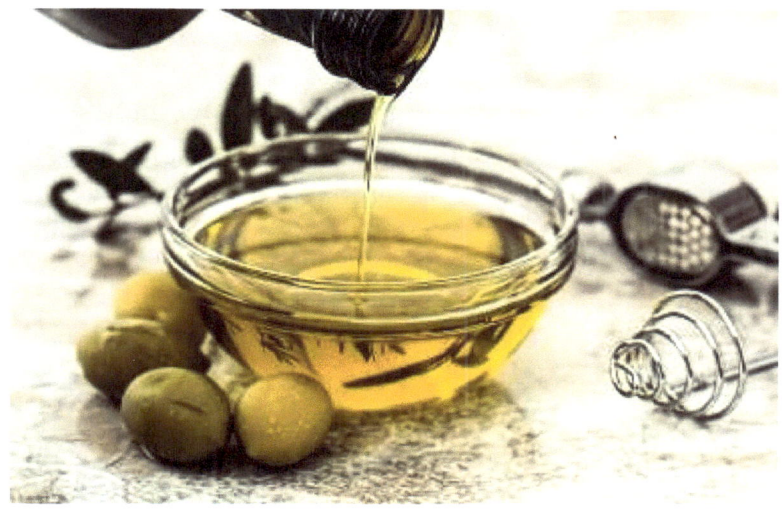

Energy is a ubiquitous term. You might want to learn a thing or two about it even if you're not a physicist. While you're reading this, you're burning some calories. Calorie is the term for unit of energy. So you hear people saying store or burn calories. They mean either you're storing or using up energy.

There are three sources of energy, all taken from food, because we're not autotrophs. The main source of energy is carbohydrates. The other two sources are protein and fats. You should consume these three macronutrients in varying amounts for proper functioning – as said previously at about 50% carbs, 30% protein and 20% fats.

While you may have been told that carbs are the staple energy source, you probably don't know that fat provides energy as well. There are certain types of diet programs based on fat as the chief energy source.

So let's talk about fat.

Popular health science has demonized fat. Doctors have blamed it for heart disease. What you must know is that it is actually an important nutrient. It cushions your internal organs. It serves as a protective layer of neurons. It serves as a vessel for certain vitamins. The vitamins A, E, D and K are all fat-soluble meaning if you are not consuming enough fat, these vitamins go through your digestive system intact and give you no benefit.

The human body is good at storing fat. We turn excess calories into fat for future use. We're still wired to store up energy in case of famine.

Anyway, there are different types of fat:

- Saturated fat. Animal fat is saturated. While it is not necessary to learn the molecular structure of saturated fats, they can be recognized by a single feature: they are solid at room temperature. The fat in meat, eggs, and milk are saturated.

- Unsaturated fat. It comes as monounsaturated or polyunsaturated fat. It's primarily found in plants. Its chief feature is lower melting point, which means it remains liquid in the kitchen. Olive oil, one of the healthiest types of fat, is unsaturated.

- Trans fat. Processing of unsaturated fats results in trans-fat. Basically a product of food processing, trans fat carries the same reputation as saturated fat. You have to consume them in minute amounts.

Fat as Energy Source

Fat is energy dense. Among the three macros, it has the highest calorie density. In other words, have the same amount of carbs, protein, and fat, and the last one gives you the highest amount of calories. A gram of fat has 9 calories. That makes it an excellent energy source. A pound of fat packs about 3,600 calories.

However, under ordinary situations your body is not programmed to burn fat. It burns glucose for energy. Excess fat is usually stored in the adipose tissue. Your body turns to this fat storage during endurance activities. When you're running a marathon, your body burns fat alongside glucose at some point.

The nature of fat and its digestion is the chief impediment to its metabolism for energy. It takes quite a while to digest fat. While carbs stay in the gut for 2-3 hours before breaking down into glucose, fat stays there for 6-8 hours. Imagine having to wait that long before your body can actually have its energy supply.

Just as it takes a long time to digest fat, it also takes a long time to convert it to energy. Tapping into your fat stores for energy is an inefficient business. That's why your body doesn't see it as a chief energy source. Your body needs more oxygen to convert fat to energy than it does when converting glucose to energy. There simple is no other mechanism where you can use fat to fuel your activities.

Carbs to Fat?

The thing is, your body likes to convert stuff to fat. Take for instance carbs. After turning carbs to glucose, your body cells gobble it up and return what's left to your liver to be used in the times of the day when your sugar goes low. If you're eating more calories than what you need for the day and much of that is carbs, your liver turns excess glycogen to fat. Your body is actually very good at doing this.

Stored fat gets used up only during times of emergency. Back in the day, stored fat is the energy source during times of famine. Your body turns to fat when carbs are scarce. Certain types of diets (i.e. Atkins and paleo) rely on high dietary fat, albeit healthy types of fat.

Caffeine and Energy

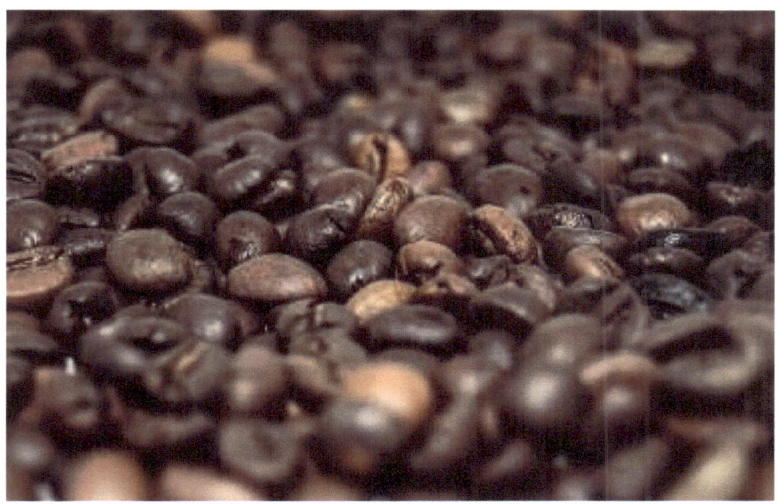

Have you noticed that you feel up and about after a cup of coffee but listless a few hours after? Perhaps you don't. If so, keep reading.

Articles about coffee abound. There's also a ton of research done to determine the health effects of coffee. It has pros and cons. Its antioxidant content is one of the reasons people drink it guilt-free.

But coffee is never potent without its caffeine content. Caffeine is like the double-edged sword in your favorite brew.

More than half of the Americans don't really pay much attention to what caffeine does. Drinking coffee is much a culture. The nutritional value is not much of an issue. Besides, it's part of people's morning routine. It's almost instinctive, a habit.

Caffeine, unlike sugar and fat, never really got a bad reputation, because there's research saying it protects you against dementia. The antioxidants in coffee may also protect you from certain types of cancer.

Plus, caffeine is fashionable. It's a stimulant, but nobody thinks of it as a drug. A cup of smoking coffee inspires images of hip, smart, and happy friends around a cocktail table. It's not like alcohol that conjures images of inebriates. But beyond all the good things that you can think of caffeine are the downsides.

Caffeine is better known as a stimulant. It's quickly absorbed in the body and affects the central nervous system. It stimulates the pituitary gland to release a hormone that activates the adrenal glands' stress response. The adrenals then release adrenaline and cortisol. Normally, your body releases these hormones in response to stress. These chemicals use up your resources, temporarily elevating your alertness and energy levels to either "fight" or "run away."

However, without imminent danger, these hormones are simply a nuisance. They only tax your body and use up calories and nutrients within the short period that they take effect. This effect is fast. Half an hour after drinking your morning brew, you'll start feeling the effects. You feel great, awake, happy, and energetic. This can last for a few hours.

But what goes up must come down. Perking you up comes with a price. Your fuel gets used up. As caffeine's effects wanes, your energy, alertness, and mood plummets. Yes, the stimulant perks you up and lets you down. Notice why you seem to need another cup of coffee after a few hours.

People who have been addicted to caffeine drink three or more cups of coffee a day just to stay awake and be able to do their tasks.

Habitual drinking of caffeine-laden drinks eventually takes a toll on the adrenal glands. Occasional caffeine ingestion doesn't affect the adrenals. They may function properly, react promptly to caffeine. Frequent stimulation of these glands cause them to go weak. At some point, they no longer react like they used to.

Weakened adrenals mean less cortisol and adrenaline produced, and that in turn means you feel the effects less. You're no longer as perked up by coffee as you were. During this phase, people think their tolerance to caffeine has increased. So they drink more coffee, thus compromising their already compromised adrenals.

In 2005, researchers studied the effect of different doses of caffeine. Subjects were divided into three groups. One group was given zero caffeine. Another group was given 300 mg of caffeine. The third group, 600 mg. After six days, the researchers gave them caffeine-laden coffee in the morning and afternoon and consequently measured their cortisol response.

The findings were predictable. The first group experienced the largest increase in cortisol. That suggested that their adrenal glands were working just fine. The other groups saw lower to almost no cortisol increase at all.

Getting rid of coffee is one of the hardest things to do. Caffeine is addictive. Stopping causes nasty headaches and lethargy that won't go away for a few days. But giving it up may be just what you need.

If you want to recover from adrenal fatigue, giving up coffee is one of the things to consider for adrenal rehabilitation.

The benefits and risks of coffee is still a matter of debate. But one thing is for sure. It's not necessary in your diet. It's not something that you need. There are certainly other things that replicate its stimulating effects. Exercise, for instance, can perk you up just like caffeine does without the adverse effects.

You can choose to withdraw from coffee gradually, taking less of it by the day. Once you turn away from it completely, you will notice more consistent energy throughout the day.

7 Foods That Rob You of Energy

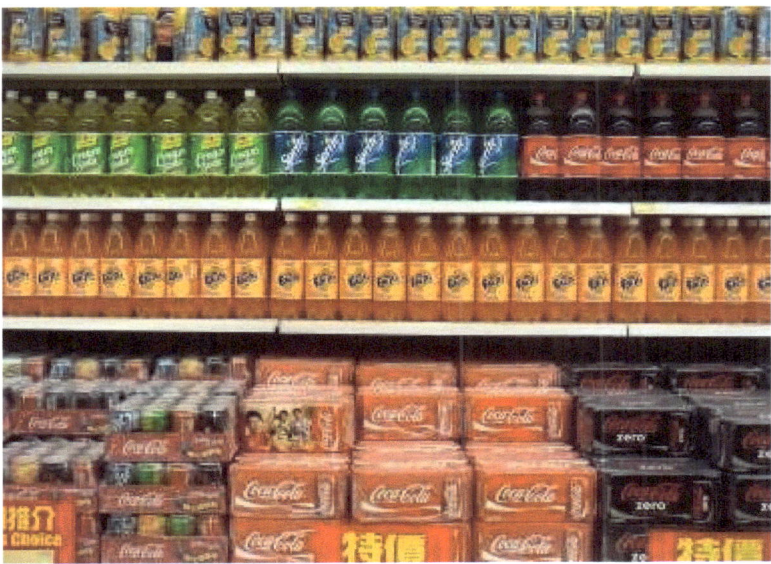

Eating should provide you energy. It should replenish nutrients you use up and lose every day. But sometimes it does not. For some reason, you feel depleted of energy, sluggish, and drowsy even if you had enough sleep or you ate enough food.

Most people don't realize how much their diet impacts their lives. What you put into your body affects not only your health but also your ability to function as an organism. Many types of food, no matter how satiating they are at first, have a peculiar way of robbing you of energy. It's ironic. Why would a meal rob you of energy? It's supposed to give you energy. But that's not always the case. That's why you have to identify these items that do the opposite.

1. Orange Juice

   Orange juice seems good, especially if you aren't
   prone to hyperacidity. It has lots of vitamin C. But if
   you haven't noticed, you feel drained a few hours
   after downing a glass of orange juice. You don't even
   realize it. Maybe you just need a nap. But what does
   an innocent orange juice have to do with it? Well, it's
   rich in fructose. This gets worse for products with
   added sugars or artificial flavors. Fructose is a simple
   sugar. It's like glucose with only a slightly different
   chemical structure. It easily gets passed into your
   body and quickly raises your blood sugar but will
   eventually leave you drained as insulin kicks in and
   drives glucose into your cells.

2. Soda

   Carbonated drinks are probably the nastiest human
   invention ever. They look cool. They look hip. A can of
   soda lures you easily when you're thirsty. You
   probably prefer it to plain water. Soda's sugar content
   is its evil head, though. It has lots of sugar. A habit of
   ingesting this sugar raises your risk of type 2
   diabetes. But you may not have to wait too long to
   feel the insidious effects of sugar. Wait for about two
   or three hours after you've gulped your soda. Watch
   out for the cravings for sweets, hunger, and
   drowsiness.

3. Coffee

   Coffee on its own isn't so bad. It's rich in antioxidants, but you may opt for green tea if it's the antioxidants you're after. Caffeine in coffee is the double-edged sword. It stimulates your central nervous system right away. It activates your stress hormones. The combined effect is you feel energized and alert shortly after you finish your cup. The catch is, it's all temporary. Within the short span of time when caffeine boosts you up, it uses up your energy reserves and leaves you drained soon. This is why coffee perks you up but then lets you down soon.

4. Fruit smoothies

   Smoothies are delicious easy-to-prepare drinks for people who are dieting. Done the wrong way, however, they are a recipe for unpleasant energy fluctuations. Fruit smoothies are high n fructose, and we already told you why fructose isn't so good. Just grab a banana or make a salad.

5. White bread

   It's all about the glycemic index. White bread is made up of refined starches. Thus, it has a higher glycemic index than wholegrain or whole-wheat bread. In other words, it quickly raises your blood sugar. You know what happens when you quickly raise your blood sugar. Your insulin rushes in. Soon, your sugar levels go down, and you feel hungry and tired.

6. Bagels

   Bagels are just like white bread. They are full of refined carbs. Have you heard of empty calories? That's what these food types are. They pack calories but have little nutritional value. They just leave you hungry after an hour or two. Next thing you know, you're grabbing another piece of bagel just to keep yourself feeling full.

7. Turkey

   But why? Turkey looks, smells, and tastes good! It's rich in amino acids, particularly in one that helps you sleep. Tryptophan is an amino acid that your body uses to make serotonin. Serotonin is a neurotransmitter that does a lot of things. One of them is to help you sleep. That makes tryptophan good at night when you're just about to nod off. In the middle of the day, it's not. Now you have an idea why people are tired after Thanksgiving.

Final Thoughts

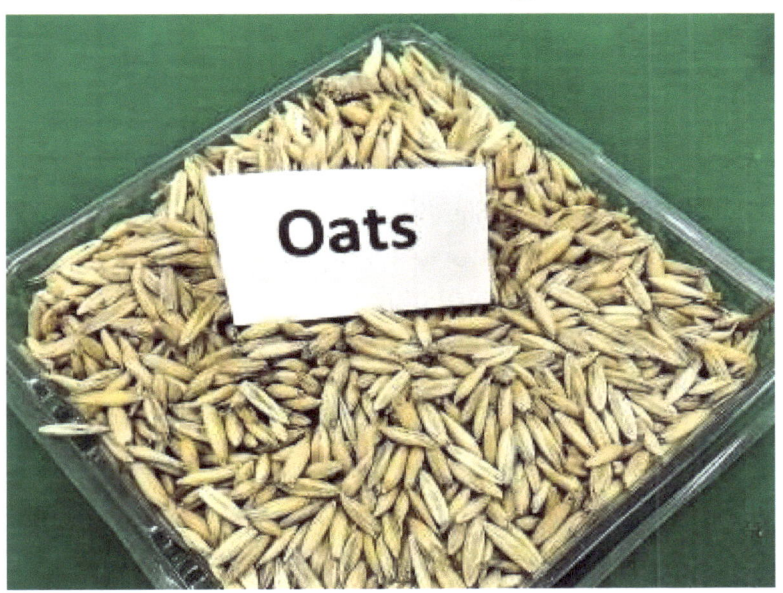

Nutrition has its crucial role in fitness. You cannot expect to see results no matter how hard you work out at the gym if your diet is crappy. Checking to see that you are getting the three macronutrients in the right proportions is an obligation you shouldn't disregard. Eat enough protein, healthy fats and carbs.

Speaking of carbs, it's important to choose the right carbs for a number of reasons. Carbs fuel your workouts. Your body gets energy from carbs, so getting enough of them means getting your fuel stores replenished every time. That way, you'll have energy for your workout and after.

All right, so when should you eat?

Let's review how long it takes for carbs, protein, and fat to digest. Your digestive system takes 6-8 hours to turn fat into fatty acids, 3-4 hours to turn protein into amino acids, and 2-3 hours to turn carbs into glucose. So you see why carbs are superior to the others in terms of fueling you.

Low GI Carbohydrates

Carbs with low glycemic index take a longer time to digest than carbs with high glycemic index. You must be wondering why the glycemic index matters. It matters because your body needs a steady supply of glucose. Only low GI carbs can provide that. High GI carbs cause spikes in glucose followed by rapid decrease, something you don't need when working out. A steady stream of glucose is what you need during and after working out. The sugar spike and crash that high GI carbs provide isn't what you need.

Your pre-workout snack should include the following carbs. Of course, don't eat them all at once. Have one type today and another tomorrow.

Oats. The fiber in oats is your best friend. It delays the digestion of carbohydrates, thus releasing glucose into your bloodstream at a slow, steady pace. Again, you need a steady supply of energy during workout.

You don't need the spike-and-crash phenomenon that happens with simple carbs. Oats also contain Vitamin B-complex, which help convert food into fuel.

Wholegrain bread. Superior to white bread, wholegrain bread, is complex carbohydrates. It's recommended for a number of reasons. It has higher fiber content. It has low glycemic index.

You can make wholegrain bread sandwiches with chicken or hard-boiled eggs or turkey.

Bananas. They are not only rich in good carbs but also in potassium. They are great if you're working out in the morning.

You should eat two or three hours before your workout. Your muscles need fuel in order to function at their best. If you work out on empty stomach, you're running a risk of depleting your fuel stores fast. Fasted workouts have their role in fitness, but it's not for everyone. If you're like most mortals, fueling your workouts is your best bet for optimal performance and gains.

What are the benefits of eating before working out?

Better Performance

Eating 2-3 hours before your workout fills up your glycogen stores. Imagine driving on nearly empty tank. It's not going to get you too far.

The same thing happens when you work out with less glycogen in your body. Your muscles just won't be able to handle the same intensity and will most likely succumb to lower fuel stores. Your progress stalls. Worse, your performance may decline, sabotaging your gains.

Muscle Gains

Protein isn't the only thing needed in muscle growth. You need carbs, too. While protein is needed to build muscles. You need carbs for energy and glycogen storage. Running low on carbs puts your body on calorie deficit. You cannot gain muscle and progress in your workouts on calorie deficit.

Your body just needs extra calories if you want to gain muscle and gain strength.

Prevent Muscle Breakdown

Not getting enough carbs is a recipe for muscle breakdown, and that's not what you need, right? Enough carbs means you give your muscles enough fuel to keep them from turning to their own protein to keep themselves working. The protein in your diet must be used up for rebuilding torn muscles, not provide energy. Providing energy is a function of carbohydrates.

Your pre-workout meal or snack should be balanced. Don't just consume carbs. Make sure you're also getting enough protein and micronutrients, such as vitamins and minerals. Keep in mind that pre-workout and post-workout meals should be part of an overall healthy diet.

About the Author

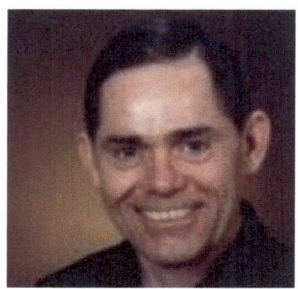

I grew up in Central Minnesota, where my parents owned and operated a fishing resort. Once out of high school I tried a couple of semesters of college, only to quit halfway through the Spring term; I decided at that time that college wasn't for me.

Then I decided to follow my father's previous occupation as an auto mechanic. I graduated from a two-year of vocational training course and worked as a mechanic for five years. While in vocational training, I decided to join the National Guard where I eventually ended up working full-time for 32 years.

So how does all of this relate to writing? In ore of my leadership schools, the instructor, who was an English teacher at a juvenile detention center, presented writing to me in a whole new way - a way that started to develop my interest in working with words.

I eventually went back to college on the GI Bill while I was working and earned my Bachelor's degree in Business Administration. Taking a class or two per semester at night and on weekends took me seven years to complete my degree.

Fast forward about 40 years and I now have published over 75 books on Amazon for Kindle, CreateSpace and other publishing platforms.

Besides my own writing, I also ghostwrite ebooks, reports, articles, blogs and do Kindle conversions for clients on a variety of topics.

Today my wife and I are retired from our careers and live in Gold Canyon, AZ. I now write as a retirement business where you'll find me happily sitting in my office typing away on my laptop as I work on my next book or ghostwriting project . . . that is if we are not traveling on a cruise ship - our new-found mode of travel.

www.ingramcontent.com/pod-product-compliance
Lightning Source LLC
Chambersburg PA
CBHW040313010626
45792CB00022B/282